What You Need to Know About Building Muscle Mass:

Tips & Strategies from 10 Top Trainers

United Print Publishers

DISCLAIMER:

This book is an educational product that provides general health information. The materials in What You Need to Know About Building Muscle Mass: Tips & Strategies from 10 Top Trainers are provided "as is" and without warranties of any kind either express or implied.

AS AN EXPRESS CONDITION TO USING THE INFORMATION IN THIS BOOK, YOU MUST AGREE TO THE FOLLOWING TERMS. IF YOU DISAGREE WITH ANY OF THESE TERMS, DO NOT USE THE INFORMATION IN THIS BOOK. YOUR PARTICIPATION IN ACTIVITIES MENTIONED IN THIS BOOK MEANS THAT YOU ARE AGREEING TO BE LEGALLY BOUND BY THESE TERMS:

This book's content is not a substitute for direct, personal, professional medical care and diagnosis. None of the advice, diet plans, or exercises mentioned should be performed or otherwise used without clearance from your physician or health care provider. The information contained within is not intended to provide specific physical or mental health advice, or any other advice whatsoever, for any individual or company and should not be relied upon in that regard. We are not medical professionals and nothing in this book should be misconstrued to mean otherwise.

There may be risks associated with participating in activities mentioned in this book, for people in poor health or with pre-existing physical or mental health conditions. Because these risks exist, you should not participate in such diet plans if you are in poor health or have a pre-existing mental or physical condition. If you choose to follow any advice within this book, you do so of your own free will and accord, knowingly and voluntarily assuming all risks associated with such activities.

Facts and information are believed to be accurate at the time they were published in this book. All information provided is to be used for informational purposes only. Products and services described are only offered in jurisdictions where they may be legally offered. Information provided is not all-inclusive, and is limited to information that is made available. Such information should not be relied upon as all-inclusive or accurate.

You agree to hold United Print Publishers, its owners, agents and employees harmless from any and all liability for all claims for damages due to injuries, including attorney fees and costs, incurred by you or caused to third parties by you, arising out of the fitness and diet plans discussed in this book.

Testimonials, case studies, and examples within this book are unverified results that have been forwarded to us by the interviewees featured in this book, and may not reflect the typical reader's experience, may not apply to the average person, and are not intended to represent or guarantee that anyone will achieve the same or similar results. You should always perform due diligence and not take such results at face value. We are not responsible for any errors or omissions in typical results information supplied to us by third parties.

DEDICATION

This book is dedicated to all the incredible professionals and companies who took the time to submit content for this book. It has been a pleasure working on the production of this book with each of you. The time you have all taken and the high quality content you have all shared has truly gone above and beyond anything we could have ever expected when we first set out to publish this book. Thank you to everyone who made this possible.

CONTENTS

ACKNOWLEDGMENTS

terraFITNESS
Sol Perry Music And Fitness, LLC
Energy Fitness
X Gym
Private Fitness Coach
Urban Pump Personal Training Studio
Trophy Fitness
San Diego Strength and Conditioning
Taylor Carpenter Personal Training LLC
Aum Training Center LLC

Thank you to the following fitness experts who without their contributions and support this book would not have been written: Terra Brozowski, Sõl Perry, Tonya Tittle, PJ Glassey, Steven Lane Weingarten, Gregg Hoffman, Kurt Chacon, Kyle Boggeman, Taylor Carpenter and Chris Carreiro

INTRODUCTION

If you've ever spent any amount of time strolling through the "Fitness & Nutrition" books section, at your local book store, you've probably noticed one thing: There sure are a lot of books on the subject of building muscle and eating healthy. While this large amount of information on the subject may seem like a good thing, it could also be the one thing that keeps you from taking action towards your personal fitness and nutrition goals.

As you're probably aware, the fitness and nutrition industry is a multi-billion dollar industry. There are thousands upon thousands of people who rely on you to buy the next fitness book, exercise gadget, or DVD that hits the store shelves or the late night TV airwaves. Unfortunately, in this profit-driven world known as the fitness and nutrition industry, one priority gets lost: Getting real results for the end-user. You see, if one of these multi-million dollar companies actually produced a gadget or DVD that enabled everyone to be in the best shape of their lives forever, you wouldn't need to buy their products anymore - and that's exactly what they don't want to happen!

So what does this mean for you? Should you just throw in the towel and give up on any and all information out there? Of course not. You do, however, need to be more selective in where you get your information from.

The goal of this book was to interview real personal trainers who really train clients each and every day of their professional lives.

When we produced this book, we set out to find real world experts and that's exactly what we got. Our biggest challenge was getting these personal trainers to break away from their busy schedules of training their clients, so that they could actually share their advice in this book. The trainers who have contributed to this book "walk the walk", and the content they've provided, in the following chapters, reflects their true knowledge and expertise. So, without further ado, we present to you, the real world expert interviews!

United Print Publishers

1 TERRAFITNESS

Pittsburgh, PA

"Answers Provided by Terra Brozowski"

Our mission at terraFITNESS is to bring the best private training experience possible to every client.

Everyone has individual goals, and we will work together to meet them. We talk to each of our clients to understand their strengths, weaknesses and limitations. We then design a personal training program based on this information. We help our clients achieve, maintain, and even exceed what they once thought was impossible. Through an approach based on a healthy diet, cardiovascular endurance, strength training and core conditioning, we make fitness a fun and exciting part of your life.

The training team at terraFITNESS comes from a varied background. We strive to make fitness fun and enjoyable. Our team utilizes the latest in sports science research along with years of experience to get you in the best shape of your life.

How many days can/should a person work out in a week?

Depending on your goals and how much time you have available, anywhere from 4-5 days a week would be ideal. You can mix in cardio and strength training, alternating between upper-body and lower-body days. Then add in a day for stretching and rest. One of the key aspects of fitness is not to run your body into the ground. Give it at least 1-2 rest days a week for optimal performance during your workouts.

What is some advice you can give a person with a busy schedule who wants to start exercising?

I strongly recommend mornings. When you work out in the morning, your body feels ready to take on the day, you are energized and you can focus on the rest of your day. Also, you won't be dreading the workout after a long work day, or using the excuse that you cannot get away from work!

However, if you know for sure that mornings won't work for you, you can try doing 30 minutes of an intense workout. I like to do HIIT (Highly Intense Interval Training) when I'm short on time, but want to get a good sweat on. You can start by warming up for three minutes, then going for a 30-second sprint, with a one minute recovery period. Repeat this 10-15 times before ending with a five minute cool down. You can do this 1-2 times per week depending on your fitness level. If you're a beginner, try once a week with your recovery intervals at a fast walking speed.

HIIT also causes your body to burn calories long after your finished working out. This is because your body takes in extra oxygen after the workout to help restore your body to its normal levels. Because this is taxing on your metabolism, it needs more energy (read: calories) to do this.

For someone who is just starting a work out plan; is having planners, schedules, calendars, etc. more or less effective in helping getting and staying motivated and determined to their work out?

It depends on the kind of person you are, but I would say treating your workout like an appointment will make you a lot less likely to skip it. Planners can also help you set goals, and stick to them. For example, if you want to lose one pound per week, mark it in your calendar! It'll be a weekly reminder to stick to your goals, which will keep you on track in the long run.

How many reps are advisable for building strength?

For general fitness, the recommended rep range is between 10-15, with the last three being difficult to perform. It is important to note that the last three are not impossible! If you're looking to build more strength, you want to lift a weight where you can only complete 6-8 reps.

How fast or slow should someone perform reps?

Repetitions should be performed slowly with good form. For general fitness, the rule of 3:1:1 applies. It means 3 seconds in the eccentric phase, 1 second in the isometric phase, and 1 second in the concentric phase. Let's break this down a bit: the eccentric phase is the lengthening phase. Think of the muscle as a slinky: this is the phase where the slinky is elongated, and is getting ready to spring into its shortened size (concentric phase). The isometric phase is where there is no joint movement, but the muscle is still contracting. What follows is one second in the concentric phase: the shortened phase. This phase releases the energy built up in the eccentric phase, and is used to overcome the resistance (weight) that is being applied.

What are the factors that affect the duration to build body muscle?

There are a few factors which are in our control, such as diet, weight lifted in a session, and how often we work out. If you are looking to add muscle, you'll need to make sure that you're taking slightly higher protein levels than the average person. The American College of Sports Medicine in conjunction with the Academy of Nutrition and Dietetics recommends 1.2-1.7g/kg of bodyweight. For example, if a 150lb person was looking to put on muscle, they would need to eat between 81.82-116g of protein per day. That individual would also be performing intense workouts where they would perform 6-12 repetitions at a weight where the last three repetitions were challenging, but not impossible. These sessions could happen 2-3 times per week, with at least 24-48 hours of rest in between, to allow for muscle recovery.

One factor we cannot control is genetics. We all have something called a genetic potential, which determines that amount of weight we can lose, and the amount of muscle that an individual can put on. Signs of approaching the genetic potential are a decrease in results in spite of proper nutrition, workouts, and rest.

Should someone go to a gym daily to build body muscle?

Building muscle is a marathon, not a sprint. If you go to the gym every day, you shred your muscles every day, and they have no time to recover. Intense daily exercise can lead to injury and over-training, which will set you even farther back from your goals. This is why rest days that include complete rest, foam rolling, stretching, or yoga are all good options to balance out your lifting program.

For people who are always tired, would exercising make them feel like they have even less energy?

On the contrary, people tend to have more energy with a regular exercise routine! This is because their bodies start properly using fuel for energy, and their hormones begin to regulate themselves. Couple a regular exercise routine with a balanced diet and you're golden!

Are warm-ups necessary to do before starting with gym work outs? Why or why not?

A warm-up is necessary for the body to prepare for exercise. It gets the blood flowing to all of the muscles, which makes them literally warm up and loosen. The warm-up also allows your body to prepare for the physical demands of exercise by pumping adrenaline into your system. A good warm-up can be 3-5 minutes of walking at a pace where you can still have a conversation, but not without pausing for a second to catch your breath.

What are some of the biggest mistakes people make when they start an exercise program?

One of the biggest mistakes is starting off too intensely. It sounds ironic, but some people start a program and begin going full-throttle soon afterwards. This quickly leads to a burn-out and sometimes injury, which can make exercise unenjoyable and also deter results. Injuries take time to heal, which means time away from the gym. It is important to approach an exercise program knowing that results come with time and effort and that it can sometimes take a few months to see major results.

The other big mistake is thinking that you can out exercise a bad diet. Unless you're working out twelve hours a day, which is NOT recommended, you need to fuel your body according to your goals. This means balancing carbohydrates, fats, and proteins so that your body has enough fuel to get you through your workouts, and to recover from those workouts. A balanced meal could look like two scrambled eggs and some fruit or toast. Something like a Greek Yogurt with low-sugar granola and berries, chicken with a sweet potato and a side salad, even a steak with some veggies would do.

Not only is it important to balance out those three macronutrients, but it is also important not to overeat these healthy foods. Even though they are healthier, your body doesn't look at calories from an apple and treat them differently than the same amount of calories from something else. This means that you need to have some idea of how many calories you're taking in, otherwise your efforts in the gym will be wasted. In order to lose weight, you need to create a deficit of 500 calories a day through diet and exercise. This can look like a 30-45 minute sweat session a day combined with one less glass of wine, or one less snack per day.

Do personal trainers normally work with clients who are only free during the weekends or during off-hours? What's typical in terms of when personal trainers are available?

Trainers tend to be as available as they can be. We want to help you! Most trainers offer sessions before 9-5 hours, and try accommodate their schedule to when their clients are free. They may also have a few weekend hours available as well, but they will go over their availability with you when you meet them to discuss a training schedule.

Contact Info:
Terra Brozowski

terraFITNESS

Pittsburgh, PA

412-901-3646

www.terra-fitness.com

2 SOL PERRY MUSIC AND FITNESS, LLC

Louisville, KY

"Answers Provided by Sõl Perry"

Sol Perry Music & Fitness is unlike any other training center. Sol Perry lost 120lbs and founded the company in 2012 in Louisville Kentucky after his mother was diagnosed with Terminal lung cancer. His brother being born severely physically and mentally disabled, Sol made it his life mission to help others feel better, look better, move better and with less pain, finding their own unique path to health and wellness through proper nutrition and exercise. One of the top trainer studios in the country, Sol and his wife have lost over 200lbs together and have a unique insight on what it feels like to be uncomfortable in your own skin. Sol wins trainer of the year every year for the City of Louisville and has helped raise over $500,000 for lung cancer and special

Olympics being active in the community. Sol trains folk from 16 - 77 in a variety of settings, private, semi-private, online/ remote and corporate consultations with an astounding success rate 6 days a week. Many clients come to Sol not even being able to squat without pain, some being cancer patients, organ transplant, diabetic, and many other health challenges. We specialize in everyday folk with total transformations from the ground up, but we also train athletes from amateurs to the pro level. Over 400 before and after photos of "real" people successfully getting "real" results. Too many trainers fail to see the most important part of training... actual quantifiable results you can see in pictures, count on the scale and feel in everyday life.

When is a spotter needed for exercises?

A spotter is generally needed on movements like the back squat, various presses and at times, chin ups and pull ups. Any movement where the load is over a client's head like "skull crushers". It keeps the clients safe, gives a feeling of security and allows them to hit the proper rep/sets/tempo on the movements. On the chins and pull ups, it's more of an assistance... helping them execute the movements with the correct engram (movement pattern). Nothing beats a proper spotter and it can be the difference between life and death and reaching your goals. If you get injured during "ego lifting", you cannot train and progress is stalled. I do not recommend forced reps spotting. Force reps are a very advanced technique and for your average gym going totally not needed to make continual progress. If anything, they derail progress and give the client a false sense of strength and stability. Full ROM with proper pacing, tempo, breathing and bracing should be the focus. A good coach will cue from the head down and make the client feel secure. Too many trainers are busy on their cell phones when they should be attending to their clients. Statistically, the bench press has the highest rate of injury and must be spotted at all times.

How does someone know how hard to push themselves when they're working out?

Use the PRE scale (Perceived rate of exertion scale) for each workout to track progress. An easy to follow rule is that the last two reps of the working sets should be challenging, but not so much where you are grinding the reps or hitting failure. Another great test is the overhead squat assessment. It will allow the trainer to see any muscle imbalances or inhibitions. Those should be fixed in the first phase of training.

If someone has just recently had surgery, can they lift weights or workout? What should be taken into consideration in these situations?

Firstly, they should be released by their Doctor before exercise. After that, asses the client with a movement screen and the Physical Activity Readiness Questionnaire (PAR_Q). Any red flags - refer out! A good trainer will have a solid referral network and could include the following – Physical therapist, Active release specialists, Muscle activation specialists, Chiros, Osteos, Dry needling, sports massage. No trainer can do it all on their own, nor should they try to. Having a network of trusted health and medical professionals is something to look for in a good trainer. The clients' well-being should always come first. A good soft tissue practitioner is a gold mine to have on your team; ART, MAT and NKT are on the leading edge and can do amazing things to boost progress and keep the client moving towards their goals. If you help "fix" something like a painful shoulder, hip, or knee for a client, they will stay with you as more trust will have been earned. Too many just chase endless PRs' with their clients and fail to see the overall health picture. Not everyone wants to be a powerlifter or bodybuilder. Many just want to feel and look better with less pain. Do not place your personal goals and interests upon your clients, everyone's path is unique and is a very personal journey.

Is it possible to lose fat and gain muscle at the same time? If so, how can this be done effectively?

Yes, it absolutely is! This is the holy grail of fitness for many to lose fat and gain lean mass at the same time. It has to be a combination of a proper diet strategy with things in place when the client falls off, proper training with the correct intensity and volume cycled properly, and supplementation to support the hormonal profile. If you over train or under train, it will all fall apart. The client will need to be assessed to test the work capacity and full nutritional profile. The Depaul University Fatigue questionnaire is a good resource to begin with. If the client is in adrenal fatigue, their progress will be greatly hampered. Adrenal fatigue is an epidemic in America. You must have the supporting nutrients in place to address any concerns per individual. A 20 year client will have a much different approach than a 50 year old.

What are some simple things people can do in their day to day routines, besides working out, to see results faster?

There's an old saying that goes: "you cannot outwork a bad diet" and this still holds true today. You will only spin your wheels if the nutrition is not in place. Training = King, Nutrition = Queen and together you have a kingdom. A simple way to begin is to ensure proper hydration. Most people are chronically in a state of dehydration. They pound soft drinks, energy drinks and coffee all day long. Those are diuretics, which pull water away from the body. Have the client measure their water and ensure they are getting a liter of filtered water for every 50lbs of bodyweight, don't guess! Have them fill up bottles at the beginning of the day. At the end, they should all be empty. This can have a profound effect on fat loss and muscle building as well as strength, no one drinks as much water as they think they do generally. It's the foundation of all life. When you work out, you need additional water and protein to match the training variables.

Is it true that it's not a good idea to do the same exercises during each workout session? Why or why not?

The general rule for changing exercise routines is determined by the training experience in years. For example: 1 year = every 6-8 weeks. 2 Years = 4-6 weeks. 3 years = 2-4 weeks 4 years = 1-2 weeks. As you can see, there's more to it than one might think. An experienced lifter may change workouts around every 6 sessions. You will generally get much better progress by picking two goals and pursuing them in a training block. Bench press and weighted chin ups, for example, for 6 weeks with the assistance work built in to handle any muscle imbalances. The trainer must understand how to "peroidize" the clients' training, with proper de-loads and recovery weeks built in to the programming. Training without a long-term plan is hoping for the best and flying blind. You must have a plan.

After someone has reached their fitness goals, how should their workout and nutrition plan be altered if they no longer wish to build additional muscle?

After goals have been reached, you must change things. For example, if a client has reached their hypertrophy goals of getting "beach body ready", have them go on a maintenance with calories and training and enjoy their beach vacation. So, to maintain strength in the legs and upper body, for example, go for two workouts a week, 2-3 sets of 4-6 reps to keep the current strength levels up with a few assistance movements. Simply by keeping the volume down (amount of work performed), and having them at maintenance, the calories will keep them where they want to be. Then, it's time to set NEW goals. Goals can and will often change with clients, this is normal and healthy. Reach goals, set new ones. But you do not want a client in a perpetual mode of dieting (whether a bulk or a cut.) Allow the client to live a full life while maintaining the body they always wanted. Remember, it's THEIR, not OUR goals that matter. Manage their hormones with proper training, rest, and nutrition and you will keep that client for life.

What are the best foods people should eat to gain energy and why are these foods so important?

This is a very individual process. Some clients work better with carbs and protein, some with higher. If a client can wake up, eat a 100 grams of carbs and not crash two hours later, they are generally carb tolerant and will be able to handle a higher carb diet. A client that is obese and gains weight just by looking at rice may be better off being put on a lower "cycled" carb protocol to get the fat off and manage their bio metrics and lower inflammation. Carbs are our bodies' preferred fuel source, but eat too many for too long and you may end up on the obese side of things with insulin resistance. I know I did, getting to 300lbs in my early 40s. Carbs are not "evil", no macro nutrient is, but they are very drug-like in the way they affect the body and everyone is different. By adding in BCAAs, peri-workout can aid as well if going lower carb. It can take some experimenting to see what works best for the individual. My lean gain muscle building clients eat a lot more carbs than my 67 year old overweight clients. You cannot have just one tool in your tool box, keep an open mind. I had an ex professional soccer player that could not gain weight. He could wake up and eat a cheesecake and feel totally fine two hours later. If I did that, I would fall into a food coma. By upping his carbs and protein combined, with a German Volume training, we put 2 inches on his chest and his waist got an inch smaller! He is a genetic outlier, they do exist.

How can someone shock their muscles into new growth?

If progress has stalled, switch it up! Doing the same thing over and over and expecting a different result is insanity. For example, if a client has been doing a functional hypertrophy phase (6-8 reps) for a while, change it to German Body Compositioning training (15 reps with shorter rest periods). By cycling periods of intensity (load lifted) and accumulation (volume of work) can jolt the client into new gains they never thought were possible. Be sure to hit both the type 1 and type 2 muscle fibers. Too many stick to 3 sets of 10 their whole training career. Another example would be to adjust the training tempo. Lowering the weight for 8 seconds and exploding up is a great tool to utilize. The late great trainer to the stars in the 1950s-50s, "Vince Gironda", had many templates that have been proven to work. 8 sets of 8, 6 sets of 6, reverse pyramiding... He used these with Arnold, Clint Eastwood and many other well-known people over the years. Another great method is to add a 25 rep finisher at the end of a workout. For example, if doing incline press for 5 sets of 6 reps, go for a drop set of 25 reps in the last set. Keep the tool box full and use the right tool at the right time.

What types of scheduling commitments are customary when hiring a personal trainer? In other words, do people normally take things one week at a

time or are they typically asked to schedule several weeks at a time with their trainer?

Having the client buy package plans ensures that they are in it for the long haul. If you are good, word will get around. If the client has no financial accountability, they will quite easily do something to get out of coming to the training session. I have tried it many different ways. If you do not have a 24 hour cancellation policy and ask to be paid ahead training, it could all fall apart rather quickly. Aim to schedule out as much in advance as possible. A good trainer will be very busy and this will become a necessity. In an age where everyone has a $1,000 phone, $200 cable bill, and 4 big screens in the house, people will spend money on things they deem a must. Have a payment plan option for the clients that stick it out with you and discounts when they stay for longer. It shows they matter to you. A trainer is the first to go to when things get tight in the economy, plan accordingly and have multiple revenue streams... i.e. Online training, detox programs, mentorship programs, group training... and make sure they WORK!

Do personal trainers usually have insurance?

A professional trainer will. A million dollar liability policy is a solid start. This is a must in this industry if you want to be taken seriously and be a professional. If you own your own facility, you will also need additional coverage. Better to have too much than too little. It's part of being in the business and telling your clients this on day one will garner respect.

Do people really lose muscle as they get older? If so, how much muscle do they lose on average, and can anything be done to slow this process down?

Starting around the age of 40, the average person loses a pound of lean mass a year. This can have a profound effect on your vitality and life! Here is the GOOD news! Sarcopenia (age related muscle loss) and osteoporosis (age related bone loss) can be offset greatly with the proper training, diet, and supplementation. Progressive resistance training makes the bones denser and aids in gaining lean mass at ANY age. As you grow older, mobility and managing inflammation become even more important. You can fight father time a good while. Look at the late great Jack Lalanne who lived to be 96 and trained an hour a day his whole life. This was way before Arnold came to America. Jack was one of the first who advocated proper diet and training. At the age of 70, he swam handcuffed, shackled, and fighting strong winds and currents. He towed 70 rowboats, one with several guests, from the Queen's Way Bridge in the Long Beach Harbor to the Queen Mary, 1 mile. Here is my favorite Jack Lalanne quote that I still find inspiring to this day.

"Dying is easy. Living is a pain in the butt. It's like an athletic event. You've got to train for it. You've got to eat right. You've got to exercise. Your health account, your bank account, they're the same thing. The more you put in, the more you can take out. Exercise is king and nutrition is queen: together, you have a kingdom" - Jack Lalanne 1914-2011

Contact Info:

Sõl Perry

You can view many amazing transformation photos on our website

Website | www.solperry.com

Email | sol@solperry.com - Subject Line "Get Fit"

Phone | 502-718-1717

Social | https://www.facebook.com/SolPerryStudios/

Instagram | https://www.instagram.com/solperryfitness/

3 ENERGY FITNESS

Memphis, TN

"Answers Provided by Tonya Tittle"

Energy Fitness is a boutique personal training & nutrition coaching studio located in Downtown Memphis since 2002. It was voted the best boutique studio by the local Health & Fitness Magazine readers 2013-2015. Energy Fitness owner, Tonya Tittle, has a Master of Science in Exercise Science. She is a Exercise Physiologist, certified by the ACSM (American College of Sports Medicine) and a is a Therapeutic Lifestyle Educator through Metagenics. Tonya created the Energize Method of getting results for clients. She has copy written over 100 workout programs that she and her staff utilize combined with fitness assessments, goal setting, injury management, nutrition coaching, meal plans, and 30 minute semi-private personal training sessions. Energy Fitness also has an online personal training monthly subscription with a workout video library of over 500 demo exercises, followed by videos, printable workouts with pictures, healthy video recipes, meal plans and self assessment injury reports. Tonya and her staff apply the science of getting results for their clients by infusing fun and laughter to get through the tough workouts.

Is a lifting belt essential?

A lifting belt is a topic of controversy and is typically worn to avoid back strain and offers extra support to ensure or cue proper form in certain lower body exercises. I don't believe that a lifting belt is necessary for the majority of the weight lifting population. The core (which consists of abs and lower back) should be the focus of training to help an individual execute proper form in every lift. During a bicep curl for example, one should engage the abdomen to avoid swinging the weights. Also, it is important to note that, to create balance and avoid injury, it is essential to work all the planes of the body during core training. Balanced movements of the core include side bending, forward bending, back bending, and twisting.

If you're a powerlifter or bodybuilder attempting to squat or deadlift the equivalent of 4 times your bodyweight, you most likely need a weight lifting belt for some, but not all, lifts.

Should someone workout with sore muscles?

Soreness, or degrees of soreness, is relative to each individual's perception. Some people have a higher tolerance to soreness than others. There is good sore and bad sore. Bad sore is noting that the range of motion is limited. Working out the muscles while they are "bad" sore can delay the recovery process and result in injury or bad form on exercises. Some areas of the body recover at slower rates and may not need to be worked again for a few days up to a week. Working out when there is mild or good soreness can actually help flush out the lactic acid from the muscles and decrease soreness. Be sure to rest the muscles at least 24 hours between weight workouts or intense cardio intervals.

Does smoking affect someone's muscle gain?

Smoking, like drinking, affects each person to varying degrees as some can recover better than others. Smoking is an attack on the various systems of the body. In the 20th century, science showed us that an individual's health was influenced 70% by genetics and 30% by their lifestyle & environmental choices. However, they have flipped those percentages in the 21st century and are now realizing we have much more control over our health and we aren't doomed to suffer our ancestors' fate.

Smoking slows down muscle building, increases your cortisol levels and interrupts the absorption of proteins, vitamins & minerals. Smoking also wrecks the immune system; meaning you may be sick more often. This influences your progress since you might miss workouts or not be able to train at full intensity. I have trained several smokers over the years and, because of their reduced oxygen availability due to constricted arteries, they seem to move through the sessions slower, thus affecting endurance in the weight training sessions as well as high intensity interval training, which also helps build muscle.

Does weight training cause people to lose flexibility?

Flexibility varies from person to person, with some people naturally more limber or many women hyper-flexible. Weight training can cause some people to tighten in some areas and become more limber in others. During the deadlift exercise for the hamstrings and lower back, using weights to help reach beyond normal range of motion can actually help lengthen the muscle and increase flexibility, as opposed to doing a toe touch alone with an individual's body weight. Overworking one muscle group and neglecting creating balance in the others can cause a loss of flexibility. There is also the matter of static stretching versus dynamic stretching. Static stretching is holding a stretch for 10 seconds to 5 minutes which can decrease strength as much as 7% if you lift within the next 24 hours. Dynamic stretching is more of a fluid movement and ....

If someone has a heart condition, can they still lift weights to build muscle?

The heart is a muscle, which means it can get stronger and more fit with cardio and weight training. While lifting weights, it is important for every individual to not hold their breath as it can cause the Valsalva maneuver. It's a moderately forceful attempt at exhalation against a closed airway, usually done by closing one's mouth, pinching one's nose shut while pressing out as if blowing up a balloon. This maneuver can also be done while pressing heavy weights and holding your breath, thereby causing internal thoracic pressure and making the blood pressure elevate, thus stressing the heart. People with heart conditions can generally benefit from lifting weights. I have personally trained many clients with various heart conditions, ranging from arrhythmia (including tachycardia and atrial fibrillation) to mitral valve prolapse. Using the RPE (rating of perceived exertion) scale of 0-10 is a great way to estimate effort during activity along with monitoring the respiratory rate. The RPE 6-20 scale is great for cardiovascular training and closely correlates with the heart rate during exercise when you add a zero to the number given. For example, if someone says my effort level during a cardio burst is 15, then their heart rate is likely to be 150 beats per minute. This can be checked on some of the cardio machines that have heart rate monitor grips. During weight training, the RPE scale of 1-10 might be a better scale when asking about the last few reps of a particular lift or movement in combination with monitoring breathing. Keep in mind that, when using the scale as a monitor, there are over raters and under raters. Individuals taking beta blockers are typically under raters.

How do genetics affect body building?

While genetics do play a role in body building & building muscle, keep in mind that the 21st century science reversed the percentages of 70% genetics to 30% environment/lifestyle choices for a person's state of health. This means that 70% of your lifestyle and environmental choices affects your health. You are not doomed to accept the fate of obesity, fatigue or disease that your family or siblings had or have developed. Side note, we each receive our mitochondria solely from our mothers which are the powerhouses of energy in every cell, while it was previously thought we got 50% from our father and 50% from our mother in all DNA. Modern day medicine has brought about functional medicine and looking at the key factors in lifestyle choices in both activity level and nutrition can bring about optimal health. Gone are the days of just looking for pills for ills. Look to food, activity and smart supplementation for optimal health and healthy aging.

You can't speak about genetics without mentioning body types and limb length. It appears easier for shorter people with smaller lever arms to build muscle than taller people with longer lever arms. Taller individuals have to go through a longer range of motion for each exercise, making exercises such as pull ups, bench press and squats harder. Because they spend more time doing the exercises, they stress their muscles and ligaments more for each repetition.

It's becoming popular and more available to get your blood tested for different biomarkers and DNA sequencing. Epigenetics is the study of the complete set of epigenetic modifications on the genetic material of a cell, known as the epigenome. Epigenetic modifications are reversible modifications on a cell's DNA or histones that affect gene expression without altering the DNA sequence (Russell 2010 p. 475). Two of the most characterized epigenetic modifications are DNA methylation and histone modification. Epigenetic modifications play an important role in gene expression and regulation and are involved in numerous cellular processes, such as differentiation/development and tumorigenesis. The study of epigenetics on a global level has only recently been made possible through the adaptation of genomic high-throughput assays. Bottom line is that our environment and lifestyle choices, food and medicine choices, etc. can turn genes on or off and lead to various diseases.

What are the major steps you need to make in order to build body muscles?

My initial answer to this question goes back to my undergraduate studies and the basic principles of physical fitness, as listed below, as well as nutrition, which I will also discuss.

1. The Overload Principle
2. The FITT Principle
3. The Specificity Principle
4. The Rest and Recovery Principle
5. The Use or Lose Principle

The overload principle means that the body will adapt to the workload placed upon it.

The F.I.T.T. principle is a little more involved as it has lots of variables (see chart on the next page):

	Resistance Training	Cardiovascular training
Frequency	Increase the number of workout days	Increase the number of workout days
Intensity	Increase the resistance / weight	Increase pace or % of Max. Heart Rate
Time	Increase time involved in exercise or Increased repetitions.	Increase time involved in exercise
Type	Changing the exercise but still working the same area of the body	Changing the workout to a different cardio exercise. Ex. jogging to jump rope

The principle of specificity states that, if you want to improve something, you must do work specific to the goal or sport. If you want to be a faster runner, you have to do sprints. Running won't make you a better cyclist. When I start training for a kayak race, I change my weight training routine to include some weight bearing twisting exercises for both my core and lower body.

The rest and recovery principle is important because it's when your muscles rest that they recover and repair. Adequate sleep and recovery between workouts is essential. You should have at least 24 hours of rest between strength training workouts. Make sure you don't work the same muscles two days in a row. If you like to do endurance cardiovascular sessions that last more than 1-2 hours or longer, then you need to realize that your weight training sessions will be harder on the same day or on the following days as your body will not be fully recovered.

The 'use it or lose it' principle states that muscle starts breaking down within 24-48 hours from lack of use (atrophy). This explains why we lose fitness when we stop exercising. The cells within the whole body start getting rid of energy they don't need and start to decay, causing aging to occur at a faster rate. Your muscles build strength (hypertrophy) with regular use.

Nutrition & Supplementation may account for 80% of your success to building and keeping muscle. You simply can't outwork a bad diet. Building muscles is about feeding them often and properly refueling during pre-workouts with branched amino acids and post workouts with protein, preferably in the form of a protein shake (whey isolate, which is dairy based, or pea & rice protein-vegan based powder supplement). Learning your cues to successfully create habit loops that ensure continued success and adapting and changing when needed is how you can build the best body possible.

What can thin people do to build muscle?

Consistency is the #1 factor in building muscle as it can take you 3 days to start losing what it took you 3 months to build. I know from personal experience what it takes to build muscle as I was a thin kid and was often called names like Olive Oyl (from Popeye) or skinny. When thin people begin a workout program, they need to build up to the heavy weights necessary to shed the thin/skinny image and turn into a lean/hard body. The bonus is that body fat levels are naturally low, so when muscle gain occurs, a very ripped look is visible, which bigger, bulkier guys often envy.

If a thin person is completely new to weight training, there should be a period of about 8-12 weeks doing 2-3 sets of mixing up between 6-8 reps and 10-12 reps as well as negative repetitions at least once per week. This will help strengthen the joints and ligaments before going with the heavier weights in order to avoid injury and overtraining. Thin people trying to add bulk/muscle faster need to limit cardiovascular sessions to 20 minutes 3 times per week in order to not burn calories at a higher rate and thus lose some gains. These cardio bouts should follow the weight training workouts to help flush out the lactic acid from the muscles and boost recovery.

Putting muscle on, for skinny people, typically requires 4-6 workouts per muscle group to build (you can build even faster if you lift twice a day, but if you do that, you'll need to take a full recovery day at least once a week and rest for at least four hours between workouts).

So what does lifting frequently look like? One popular split that bodybuilders have been following for years that works very well is to exercise your chest and back on day one, your shoulders, biceps and triceps on day two, your legs and core on day three and then take a day of to rest. Repeat.

Mit it up by adding plyometrics/explosive reps and sets, one quarter reps, ladder reps, super slow reps, forced reps, negatives and cheating. On the cheating, it will be necessary to use the other arm to assist in getting some or all of the reps completed. Just avoid bad form.

Let's talk nutrition & supplements as it's a huge factor in successfully building muscle for thin people. Below are some key factors in adding or keeping muscle:

1.   Eat frequently (every 2.5-3 hours) and protein every meal if possible. The body can't store protein like it can fat

and carbohydrates. The average individual can typically metabolize about 40 grams of protein every 4 hours.

2.   Eat enough calories! To gain one pound per week from food consumption, you have to take in 3500 additional calories. That is 500 extra calories per day. Not eating enough calories is like trying to build a two story house with only enough bricks for a one story one.

3.   Eat meat. I personally only eat turkey and fish as my "meat" choices as I try to eat foods for my blood type, blended with a gluten-free, dairy-free Mediterranean. I eat a lot of eggs and egg whites as well as supplements with pea and rice protein shakes. In order to get enough protein each day, I add protein powder to alternative desserts (mix and freeze-cashew nut butter, coconut oil, turmeric, salt, chia seeds & powder)

4.   For calories and upping your protein intake, protein powder is important. Try not to have more than two shakes per day as there is no substitute to whole food nutrition. There is a magical 30 minute post workout window that, as we say at Energy Fitness, "Your workout isn't over until you have nutritionally supported it." If you don't want the typical gut distress that comes from eating protein powders, don't just settle for any version of protein powder. Try to choose one without added soy and corn, with no artificial sweeteners, and with added digestive aids, such as digestive enzymes and probiotics. Whey protein isolate is a good choice for those that consume dairy. For vegans or mostly

vegetarians like myself, try pea and rice protein. I use Metagenics Cardio 360 and Ultra Meal.

Other supplements that can effectively help a thin person gain muscle are:

-Amino Acids: branched chain 5 grams (1 level teaspoon) before and after workouts (pill form is better as it is - devoid of artificial sweeteners)

-Creatine: 0.3 g/kg bodyweight for 5-7 days, followed by 5 g/day.

-Carnitine: 750 mg, 2,000 mg/day, in 2 doses.

-Citrulline: 6-8 g, 30-60 minutes before exercise.

-Beta-Alanine: 2-5 g, 30-60 minutes before exercise (this supplement is best when cycled 6 weeks on and 4 weeks off)

-L-Glutamine: 5 grams before exercise

None of these supplements are a substitute for lifting frequently and lifting heavy, but they will certainly help to enhance results.

Are there ways to reduce recovery time or soreness between workouts without taking supplements?

Performing 10 minutes of moderate cardiovascular exercise immediately after a weight training session can help flush out lactic acid thereby reducing soreness and increasing recovery time. Using a foam roller, a fascial release ball, a tool or self massaging every other day after workouts can be a way to reduce recovery time and soreness between workouts. Strenuous workouts can cause adhesions to build up in the fascia, causing a limited range of motion and soreness. Stretching immediately post workouts, along with making sure to get up several times during the day and walking/ moving around, can keep the muscles warm and prevent stiffness. Getting enough rest is essential for recovery as that's when the muscles repair themselves. Nutritionally supporting your workouts can help fuel and shorten recovery after and between workouts, giving your body the nutrients it needs to bring about optimal health. Be sure to include a variety of food and try including broccoli & pineapple, which are well known to reduce inflammation and pain.

If someone reaches their muscle building goals, should they still continue to work with a personal trainer?

What often occurs when personal training clients reach their initial goals is that their goals change. They want and need the guidance to help them reach other steps on the ladder with the desire to avoid injury as they do this. There is something to be said when accountability is part of what a personal trainer offers and when there may be lots of days you won't push yourself hard enough to get the results you crave for. Great personal trainers are more like coaches and work closely, making fitness assessments to measure progress and working with the clients' bodies to change and adapt the workouts as needed.

What are some simple things people can do in their day to day routine, besides working out, to see results faster?

Get at least 7 hours of sleep every night. Reduce sugar and processed foods and go towards less ingredients, more real and whole food. In other words, no more fake food. Reducing stress can lower cortisol, which means less chance of storing fat in the abdomen area. Eat breakfast, take your lunch to work, shop for snacks to keep in your car, purse, briefcase & office. If you work from home and tend to either not eat or eat too much of the wrong kind of calories, then pack your lunch and put it in a small cooler/tote bag together with the snacks you are to eat each day as to eliminate the decision making factor when you are hungry or past hunger.

When considering hiring a personal trainer, should the client be expecting what they want out of the sessions or what the trainer thinks is necessary?

There are many different types of personalities in this world. Some people know they need to do something but aren't willing to because it doesn't fit into their lifestyle or personality. With this realization, the personal trainer needs to adapt how she/he talks or responds to each client in order to get the client to move and change so they can reach their goals. Even before a personal trainer meets with a prospective client, they ask about their goals and what they are doing now. Next, the trainer should tell them about their method of training and how they get results for clients. Ideally, the trainer asks if they want to come in for a free consultation. It is during this meeting that the personal trainer can ask the prospective client more detailed questions, show them their method of personal training in the form of a flip chart presentation with successful client pictures and stories in which they can relate, what the trainer expects from the client and vice versa. This initial interview with a prospective client needs to be an honest conversation about the motivation behind someone wanting to hire a trainer, as trainers are trying to foster a coaching environment and create new habit loops to elicit change. Fitness assessments and nutrition coaching are key to helping create a relationship that has respect and realistic goals with specific time frames. Often time, the clients look to the personal trainer as the professional to help them set realistic goals. Sometimes it's easier for someone else to see the changes that need to be made than the person wanting or needing to make them. In my experience, people often want to achieve a certain level of fitness or look, but aren't willing or don't know how much work it really takes to get there. Changing one habit per month is often a great way to start working towards the clients' goals. Too many changes too fast is overwhelming and can lead to failure for many people. Nutrition is the hardest area for most people to change as we all have to make the choice of what to eat numerous times per day.

Contact Info:
Tonya Tittle
Energy Fitness, 552 South Main
Memphis, TN 38103
Phone: 901-523-2348
Energy Fitness Online training &
Website: energymemphis.com
Supplements website: EFitness.Metagenics.com
www.facebook.com/energyfitnessmemphis
www.linkedin.com/in/tonya-tittle
energymemphis@gmail.com

4 X GYM

Seattle, WA

"Answers Provided by PJ Glassey"

The X Gyms are the Seattle area's premier one-on-one personal training facilities, specializing in high intensity workouts requiring only 21 minutes, twice a week, to achieve optimum fitness. Our advanced, safe and exclusive exercise techniques, combined with the most effective equipment available and the best nutrition guidance, produce results equivalent to about 7 hours of traditional training per week. The X Gym has clubs in Alki (West Seattle) and the Eastside (on the border of Bellevue and Kirkland).

How should people with asthma approach their workouts?

People with asthma should always warm up first and then progress slowly with their intensity level. They should back off intensity immediately as soon as they start feeling asthma symptoms coming on. If they have an inhaler, they should use it at the first sign of needing it.

Is weight lifting a good idea for people who have high blood pressure?

Weightlifting is definitely a good idea for people with high blood pressure because that will be one of the tools necessary to reduce that blood pressure. They do, however, need to avoid the Valsalva maneuver or any breath holding like that, even for a short moment. Restricted exhaling can also be harmful, so unrestricted airflow, both in and out, is necessary. This, in my opinion, is how everyone should breathe, whether they have high blood pressure or not. I always teach constant airflow, either in or out, based on what the body wants to do, regardless of whether it is during the "push" phase or "recovery" phase of the repetition.

How does a person prevent stretch marks?

There are certain moisturizers, oils and vitamin treatments that may work for some people, but there is no single treatment that works for everyone. Some people find, that no matter what they use, they still get stretch marks, because they are that kind of a person. Other people never get stretch marks, regardless of preventative measures or treatments. Gaining fat rapidly is the fastest way to stretch marks (besides pregnancy), but it can also happen with rapid muscle gain, so obviously, the way to prevent stretch marks through rapid muscle gain is to take more time and gain that muscle more slowly.

How often should someone increase the weight?

Traditional training recommends the weight should be increased if you can do 8 to 12 repetitions in good form after three or more sets. We don't do traditional training at the X Gym however, so we have a different set of rules. We just do one set in perfect form to complete fatigue, so if someone can complete all their repetitions under those parameters, we raise the weight. When we do raise the weight, we typically raise it by only 5% because the controlled way we train necessitates small resistance increases.

How can someone speed up the muscle recovery?

Good nutrition is the most important thing for muscle recovery, which includes proper hydration, since muscles are after all, about 75% water. Getting enough quality sleep is the second most important factor. Third is making sure overtraining doesn't happen. Genetic factors play a huge role in this, because people who are gifted with the right hormones tend to recover faster than "normal" people (like myself).

What is some input people should keep in mind for practicing good form during their workouts?

The last rep should look exactly the same as the first rep. Form and posture should never degrade during the set, especially in order to achieve more reps or a certain amount of weight. Concentration 100% of the time during each rep and diligent focus on form should be top priority. We take people to complete muscle fatigue and then beyond with our training style, but never at the expense of form. That last, hardest rep will look just the same as the first, easiest rep.

What does intensity mean?

Intensity can be measured in many ways, ranging from perceived exertion, to heart rate, to breathing rate, muscle fatigue, etc. The way we measure intensity is through complete muscle failure in perfect form. When someone reaches true muscle failure, their intensity is automatically maximized. There are four stages of muscle failure to work through in order to maximize the intensity. The first stage is mental fatigue, when the brain says you're done. The second stage is concentric fatigue, when you can't push the weight out anymore and you get stuck. The third stage is isometric fatigue, when you can't even hold the weight in place any longer and it slowly starts to slide back. The last stage is eccentric fatigue, when you can't even control the speed of the way it slides back. This is the highest intensity someone can reach on their own, but with a spotter and training partner assisting, you could even get past this stage. For cardio training, intensity is more about heart rate and breathing rate. Tabata interval training is a good example of high intensity cardio because each sprint segment is 100% intensity, yet each segment will slow down if this technique is done properly, showing the fatigue from the intensity.

What are the best exercises for muscle building?

Compound movements are the best for functional strength, but isolated movements are the best for bulking the muscle up. Bodybuilders incorporate both though, because compound movements are also the best for eliciting optimal hormone response for muscle building. High weight and ballistic repetitions are also useful in muscle building because that style causes micro tears which create scar tissue that is larger than the original muscle fiber. Heavy eccentric training ("negatives") is also effective at creating micro tears. Our style uses light weights and controlled repetitions, so micro tears are never experienced, hence no scar tissue is ever formed. We also do only one set to complete fatigue, taking 2 to 3 minutes for each set, instead of short, multi-set training, which is also very effective for muscle building. Needless to say, our clients are interested in muscle building, so our system is designed to strengthen, tone and define without muscle bulk.

What type of cardio should someone do that won't hinder their muscle building?

High intensity interval training is the best form of cardio for someone who is interested in muscle building. Long-duration, steady-state cardio will absolutely work against muscle building.

What should a personal trainer take into consideration when working with each individual client?

A personal trainer should always be mindful of their client's limitations, injuries and contraindications first, so their workout is as safe as possible. Second, they should learn their client's "buttons" and the things that motivate them, so they can make their experience something they will want to come back for.

If a personal trainer is always showing up late, should the client still be expected to pay for the full session? What's the customary way to deal with a situation like this?

In my opinion, if a personal trainer is ever late – even by one minute – the session should be half off. If the trainer is more than 10 minutes late, the session should be free. If this happens often, the client should simply fire that trainer. Being on time shows respect. If there is no respect, there should be no relationship. That client should find a trainer who does respect them.

How will a trainer know what program is right for their client?

A thorough health history form and goals interview should be enough for a qualified trainer to design the right program. After that, trial and error, along with constant feedback from the client will refine the program. For every exercise we do, there are dozens of other exercises that can be done to target that same muscle, so if the client simply doesn't like an exercise, they shouldn't be forced to continue with it, if the trainer is creative enough.

Contact Info:
PJ Glassey
pj@xgym.com
xgym.com
pjfit.com

5 PRIVATE FITNESS COACH

Louisville, KY

"Answers Provided by Steven Lane Weingarten"

I'm a self-employed personal trainer based in Louisville Kentucky. I specialize in contest prep for bodybuilders, physique athletes and figure and bikini competitors. I also help highly motivated "normal people" achieve their fitness goals.

Do you need to take supplements for muscle building?

No, they're not required. But a couple of inexpensive, well-researched supplements — creatine and beta-alanine — can assist with muscle building. I think they're best used to blast past a plateau.

When should a person take protein shakes? Is it necessary to? Why or Why not?

Protein shakes are not required, but they can be a convenience. There's nothing magical about protein shakes; they're just food in liquid form. Someone eating 5 or more meals daily to promote hypertrophy might occasionally find themselves time-crunched and unable to eat a solid-food meal. That's where a protein shake can prove invaluable.

Some bodybuilders believe that drinking a protein-and-carbohydrate shake while training (an intraworkout shake) can accelerate muscle building, but the science on that isn't 100% conclusive.

Can eating before you go to bed help the process of quicker muscle building?

Yes. Having an around-the-clock intake of calories and amino acids is critical to muscle building. Some super-serious bodybuilders even wake up in the middle of the night to drink a protein shake. Bodybuilders eat 5, 6 or more times daily to keep the body in an anabolic (growing) state.

Is working out at home less effective than in a gym? If so, why or why not?

It depends. Some people can motivate themselves just fine, or prefer training in solitude. Others (probably most people) do better surrounded by like-minded people who can encourage and spot them. There is most definitely something inspiring about working out in a hardcore gym amongst other people striving to better themselves.

And, it's expensive to equip a home gym with the same variety of equipment you can find in a commercial gym.

Do people really lose muscle as they get older? If so, how much muscle do they lose on average, and can anything be done to slow down this process?

Yes, sarcopenia (age-related muscle loss) is a real thing. For sedentary people, this can begin at around the age of 30. Sarcopenia accelerates in those aged 50+, with people in this age group losing around 1% of their muscle mass each year. Sarcopenia is the main cause of frailty and lack of locomotion seen in the elderly.

Resistance training is the best way to retard this process. In one study of more than 1,300 adults over the age of 50, researchers showed that resistance training increased the participants' muscle mass by an average of nearly 2.5 pounds in just five months.

How can someone bring out their abs?

Most people who lift weights have developed decent abdominals through their efforts in the gym, but their abs are obscured by a layer of fat.

Exposing abs — in other words, obtaining muscular definition, is a matter of negative calorie balance. You have to intake fewer calories than you burn, so that your body uses the stored fat for energy. The best way to achieve this negative calorie balance is though a small calorie decrease combined with a small cardio increase.

It's a waste of time doing set after set of sit-ups or other ab exercises in the belief that this will bring out your abs. Many bodybuilders with outstanding abs step onstage having done zero or very little ab work during their show preparation.

How can someone build the lower body without weights?

Sprints on a bicycle can build some impressive quads and hamstrings. Heel-to-toe walking is a great calf builder.

How should someone's age be taken into consideration when starting a new exercise program?

The older someone is, the more likely they are to have injuries, degenerative issues, or metabolic concerns that can impact their ability to train and recover from exercise.

On the other hand, a young teen or pre-teen needs to be taught to curb their enthusiasm to show off and lift weights heavy than they are ready for.

How often should someone switch up workouts?

I like clients to stick with the same program for as long as 3-4 months, gradually increasing the weights lifted and mastering the performance of each exercise. Change to a new program when you hit a plateau. The so-called "muscle confusion" principle, which claims that you have to "trick" muscles to make them grow by constantly changing exercises? There's no science to back that up. Muscles don't respond to random changes in exercises — they respond to gradually escalated stress. That means adding weight, increasing reps and/or sets, or decreasing the time between sets. Make your muscles work harder and they'll grow!

How hard should someone work each set?

Training to failure — and even beyond failure via forced reps, drop sets, and other intensity-enhancing techniques — is a great way to generate progress. However, the harder you train, the less volume you should do. If you're the type who prefers to push every set to the max, it's prudent to do fewer sets than someone who stops sets a few reps shy of failure.

What are some questions people should ask a personal trainer before hiring them?

Find out the trainer's qualifications and policies and ask if you can speak to a couple of the trainer's clients to get first-hand knowledge about the trainer's methods, personality, competence and reliability. While you're interviewing the trainer, assess how well the two of you "gel"; you're going to spend a lot of time together, so make sure that that time is enjoyable, as well as productive.

Contact Info:
Steven Lane Weingarten
kyfitnesscoach.com
flexwriter@aol.com

6 URBAN PUMP PERSONAL TRAINING STUDIO

Denver, CO

"Answers Provided by Gregg Hoffman"

Urban Pump Personal Training Studio was co-founded by Gregg and Sharon Hoffman. We offer one on one training, semi private training, and small group classes. Urban Pump exclusively uses the Hystrength(sm) fitness program developed by Gregg Hoffman. The Hystrength(sm) fitness program is so efficient that only two twenty minute workouts are needed for a fit, shapely body. Urban Pump Personal Training Studio offers online coaching as well.

When it comes to nutrition about building muscle, it seems that few experts can agree on what is a healthy diet and what is not. How can people know

which advice to take, with all of the contradictory information out there?

Everybody needs to do their own research and not take the suggestions of the fitness trainer at face value. The truth is that there are many similarities between many of the good diets out there. It is these common threads that should be the cornerstone of a healthy eating plan. Beyond that, it is a matter of tweaking the diet to how the person's body responds the best, along with his or her personal eating preference.

It is said that you should have a meal of proteins or carbs after a workout. Is that true? If so, why?

The prevailing theory is that the body is primed for nutrient absorption right after a hard workout, especially the first two hours afterward. With this, trainers assume that a meal replacement shake will create the optimal muscle building environment. Personally, I do not think ingesting a protein shake right after a workout is all that important. I stumbled on some research suggesting that the body maintains that nutrient absorption window for much longer than previously thought...up to 24 hours actually. Imagine that. A good intense workout sends the signal to the body to build muscle, and it will do so regardless of whether the trainee eats something right after the workout or not. It has plenty of resources to draw on to start the muscle building process. Unless the trainee is an athlete in training and in need of a high calorie diet, I generally recommend restraining eating anything until the trainee feels hungry. The rationale behind this approach is that, after an intense workout, the glycogen stores will be empty, thus forcing the body to rely on the fat stores for fuel. In essence, it assists in the fat burning process and the body will still gain muscle. I have been very successful with this approach.

What type of protein powder is best for muscle gain?

Most experts will say that whey protein is the best for muscle gain, and that may be true. However, the benefit, in my opinion, is negligible. There are many good protein sources that will do a good job, and I would rather encourage my clients to eat real food with a good amount of protein and healthy fats.

What is the correct way to breathe when working out and how does it help a person when lifting weights?

The conventional recommendation for breathing is to breathe in during the eccentric portion of the lift (lowering phase), and to breath out while performing the concentric part of the lift (lifting phase). It is assumed that the trainee will be able to accomplish a higher number of reps in this manner as opposed to, say, holding the breath at certain points of the set. I have no disagreements with this strategy, but I much prefer to have my clients use a short/shallow breathing technique accompanied with actually holding the breath briefly at the sticking point. My clients are able to focus much better on the performance of the lift this way, and the holding of the breath for a brief moment during the sticking point actually helps the client finish the rep.

If a particular exercise hurts, is that normal?

It depends on the hurt. The burning sensation someone experiences during a strength training exercise is a good thing. In essence, it means that the muscle is working very hard, which is the stimulus needed to make it stronger. On the other hand, if the trainee feels a sharp pain, usually close to the joint, then the trainee needs to stop the lift. Working through this kind of pain over a period of time can lead to soft tissue injuries.

What should someone do if they get muscle cramps during a workout? Should they work through it or do something else?

Muscle cramps during a workout session are rare, but it is usually a sign of dehydration or an electrolyte imbalance. Stop the exercise routine immediately and get some fluids.

Which are better, free weights or machines? Is there a huge difference and if so, why?

Better for what? Building muscle? The stimulus for building muscle is rather simple: Make the muscle work as hard as possible in a short amount of time. Realizing this, both machines and free weights can accomplish that task remarkably well. Having said that, there are unique benefits to both free weights and machines. Machines, for example, are designed to coincide the resistance curve with the strength curve of the muscle. Stated differently, the resistance will either get heavier or lighter during the range of motion to match the changing strength level of the muscle. As an example, the hamstrings will be able to produce more force when the leg is straight, and less force in the fully contracted position. If the machine does not adjust for this, the weight will be just right at the beginning of the lift but very heavy at the end. The machine's main goal is to keep that tension, if you will, constant throughout so there is no point where the muscle gets a chance to rest, nor too heavy for the muscle to complete the lift. Moreover, machines are designed to isolate a certain muscle group to force that particular muscle to work harder. However, the strengths I mentioned of machines are also the downfall of machines. By isolating muscle groups to such a degree as machines do, there are many supporting muscles that do not get very much stimulus to get stronger. A good example is the rotator cuff muscles of the shoulder joint. The primary purpose of the rotator cuff muscles is to provide stability and support for the shoulder while the chest and back muscles are working (they also create movement as well, for the rotator cuff muscles are the primary muscles used in swinging a tennis racket or throwing a baseball), and a chest press machine has a set groove throughout so the rotator cuff muscles do not have to work very hard to stabilize the shoulder. This can lead to the chest muscles getting stronger than the rotator cuff muscles, creating a muscle imbalance. In theory, this imbalance can lead to injury. Free weights, on the other hand, address this shortcoming. When performing a lift with free weights, the trainee has to both lift the weight and balance it at the same time. The smaller stabilizer muscles work much harder to accomplish this task.

Additionally, free weights offer many more exercise options than machines. Machines usually perform only one function, whereas a dumbbell can be used for many exercises that can work different muscle groups. There is one final consideration, and that is personal preference. Since both machines and free weights are capable of improving strength, it is better for the trainee to decide what he wants to use. Personally, I prefer to use a combination of free weights and machines.

What advanced techniques should someone use to build muscle?

There are many useful advanced techniques one can use to build muscle.

Here is a brief list:

Forced reps
Negative reps
Descending sets
Super-sets
Pre-exhaustion

The first three are considered set extension techniques in that they help the trainee work beyond failure/fatigue on a set. The other two are variations of a combination of sets with very short rest intervals specifically targeting a muscle group such as the legs or chest. They are very effective protocols to have in the toolbox, but the secret is in using them very sparingly. As an example, when a trainee does a set to fatigue, he may have the spotter help him with two or three more reps after the fact (forced reps) in an attempt to work harder. The truth is that one good rep beyond failure is all the trainee would need because, if he knows he will be doing multiple reps after failure, he will hold back a little on the previous reps. This will make the set extension technique less effective. It would be better if he just focused on completing one good rep after failure. The same principle applies to all of the advanced techniques. It is much better to use any one of these techniques once every other workout, and for only one body-part per workout.

What are the basic exercises to do for muscle mass?

This is a good question. Compound exercises, which are exercises that create movement around two or more joints, seem to work the best. Leg presses, barbell squats, and dead-lifts are great for building mass for the legs. Likewise, dumbbell presses or the bench press work very well for building the chest muscles. Isolation exercises such as a leg extension or cable fly do not work as well because one cannot use as heavy of resistance as with compound movements.

How can someone tell if their personal trainer's certification is legitimate?

Many, if not all of certifications will give the aspiring personal trainer a base knowledge of exercise, physiology, anatomy, nutrition and other criteria to be a competent trainer. The truth is that a certification is not what makes an exceptional trainer. I put much more value on a trainer that spent time working as an apprentice under a highly respected fitness trainer or organization through continuing education, mentoring, and studying the latest research. Moreover, testimonials have far more value in showing the competency of a fitness trainer than the certifications he may have. To put it simply, getting a certification is the starting point for the fitness trainer, but the true value is garnered through experience in the field.

How can people get motivated to get to the gym?

This is a multi-layered question and yet unique to every individual. The individual may be motivated to begin an exercise program for many different reasons, which is good, but maintaining the motivation over the long haul is the real challenge. A high percentage of people quit their exercise program after a few months, if not weeks, of starting it. I believe there are three main causes of decreased motivation. Most exercise programs require a big time commitment on a weekly basis. The results do not come along as expected. Burnout. Most exercise programs will have the trainee in the gym anywhere from 4 to 8 hours a week. The trainee will have no problem committing to this regimen at first, but it will get tiring after a few weeks. Additionally, once life starts getting in the way, say, by needing to take the kids to a play or the boss wanting the fitness enthusiast to stay late on a project, he will start missing workouts. This will throw off his whole routine and he may just give up.

The other problem is that many exercise programs really do not work very well. The trainee can spend several hours a week in the gym for some time and may lose a couple of pounds of fat. The return on investment, if you will, is not very good. This is very demotivating, and the trainee will most likely quit.

The final reason I believe that many people have a hard time staying motivated is from burnout. Spending a large amount of time in the gym working out will lead to over training. The trainee may get injured or he may simply be tired all of the time, and he will quit working out. It has been my philosophy to streamline the exercise program so that the trainee can see remarkable results with very little time in the gym. I have had great success with client motivation and retention this way. I recommend it for anybody who wants to make a lifelong commitment to the fitness lifestyle.

Do most personal trainers yell at people, like drill sergeants, to keep them motivated? What if someone wants to hire a personal trainer without being screamed at?

Ha. This question reminds me of a local personal training studio that used anger and insults to motivate the client base. The owner would refer to the women as fat bearded ladies and the men as sissies. He would also throw Twinkies at the clients when they were exercising and would put them in cages if they did not work as hard as he thought they should. It was all a gimmick, and he did have some initial success. Moreover, many trainers do use loud screaming and drill sergeant tactics to motivate the clients. Personally, I do not subscribe to this strategy. I think most people have enough negative feedback to deal with in regular life. They certainly do not need it in the gym. I much prefer to use positive reinforcement and good rapport to facilitate my clients fitness transformation. I do believe that the positive reinforcement strategy does a much better job at helping the client internalize a fitness minded lifestyle.

Contact Info:

Gregg Hoffman

President, Urban Pump Personal Training Studio

2322 Central Park Blvd,

Denver, Co 80238

303.587.0149 (cell)

gregg@urbanpump.com

7 TROPHY FITNESS

Dallas, TX

"Answers Provided by Kurt Chacon"

I provide skill, knowledge and experience to help people look better, feel better and live better through the use of exercise, lifestyle habits, and sound nutrition.

Should people bring a note pad to the gym to record their time?

Record keeping is important. That which is measured, improved. People can use notebooks and pencils, but they can also use their phones or other fitness related recording devices. The only way you can know if you're getting better is to record your results.

How much sleep does someone need for optimum muscle growth?

In my opinion, as much as one can reasonably get to. But if someone is consistently sleeping less than seven hours a night, they are probably not building all the muscle they can.

Should people stretch between sets? If so, how effective is it?

I have used stretching between sets with clients who have a specific issue or buddy area that needs attention. I have found that it does work in some cases. As to whether or not it builds flexibility generally, I have no opinion.

How can people increase testosterone naturally?

Strength train, get plenty of nutrition, which includes proteins, minerals and fats (the building blocks of hormones), get plenty of sleep, and avoid obesigens and other endocrine disruptors in our air, water, food, and products we apply to our bodies.

How does someone know if they're "over-training"?

My experience tells me that a few people over traine. Many people over reach, which is a specific goal designed to produce adaptations. Generally, results stop, the client fatigues easily, can't sleep, and may even regress with overtraining.

Should someone use the full range of motion?

What is the motion? "What is the goal" is how I respond. The range of motion is dependent upon the exercise, the intensity, the frequency, and the desired outcome. Also, the clients' anatomy and physiology also play a role, as well as any injury or limitation the client might have. Then we can discuss what a "full range of motion" is.

Do people need a trainer in a gym to perform the work outs?

Absolutely not. The client should be encouraged to do their own workouts and take responsibility for their own fitness and well-being in the gym.

What if someone is completely out of shape? What's the safest approach for getting started?

Start slowly, build consistently, and make small goals. I learned early in my career that, if you start somebody at zero, you can't hurt them.

How can a person build massive strength without getting too big?

Meditations in the body exist along a continuum. Low reps, such as one, two, or three tend to produce neurological changes without muscle hypertrophy. That is how weightlifters who weigh 135 pounds can clean and jerk over 400 pounds. The changes that result from their training are virtually all neurological.

If someone has just recently had surgery, can they lift weights or work out? What should be taken into consideration in these situations?

First of all, the nature of the surgery dictates what people can and cannot do after surgery. Also, understanding the condition of the client when they underwent surgery is important. Somebody who's been training and exercising for years and years will recover much faster and regain the ability to exercise sooner than someone who did not work out very often or at all. The directive of the physicians involved should always be made first priority.

If someone feels they are not able to build their muscles even after doing heavy workouts, what may be the cause?

I have found that people rarely have a proper nutrition to support their level of exercise. This would include the wrong mix of nutrients, the lack of nutrients, poor timing of nutrition, and nutritionally bankrupt foods. Also, exercise or failing to understand how muscle growth works may sometimes be the cause.

Contact Info:

Kurt Chacon

www.allaboutiron.org

214-533-2634

coachkurt@me.com

8 SAN DIEGO STRENGTH AND CONDITIONING

San Diego, CA

"Answers Provided by Kyle Boggeman"

Located 6346 riverdale street San Diego 92120. We prioritize strength in basic compound movements as well as intelligently placed conditioning for first time exercisers, athletes, military and law enforcement.

In resistance training, how does the ratio of weight to reps affect muscle building?

There is no clear answer to this. We know muscles can grow through 3 different mechanisms: mechanical tension, muscle damage, and metabolic stress. Any one of these mechanisms is capable of stimulating growth. Anecdotally, many strength athletes have built impressive physiques on a diet of singles, doubles and triples, primarily maximizing mechanical tension overload. Bodybuilders are known for their high training volumes (often with higher reps), maximizing muscle damage and metabolic stress. I would hazard a guess and say most successful natural physique athletes utilize all three mechanisms of growth, either through periodization, or with higher volume back-off/accessory work after strength work. My recommendation for beginners would be to focus on mechanical tension overload as the main driver of hypertrophy, but do so in a repetition range that allows you to accumulate a moderate amount of muscular damage and metabolic stress. This would mean getting stronger primarily in the 5-8 rep range for the main compound lifts. Going higher in reps often forces a tradeoff between mechanical tension and metabolic stress, and this can make getting stronger a lot harder. My feelings are that mechanical tension should be prioritized, if for no other reason than because long term strength adaptation allows a trainee to handle heavier weights for more reps later on. Once you have a solid strength base, experiment with different rep ranges and higher volume assistance work.

How can someone make sure they're not burning muscle when they're working out?

I don't think this is usually a concern, provided you aren't doing excessively long, slow distance cardio, or in a severe calorie deficit. In general, focus on strength training, progressive overload, and use reasonable training volumes. Make sure you are eating enough to recover properly from the training.

How quickly is food converted to fat or muscle mass? Is one of these made more readily than the other?

Your ability to convert food to muscle or fat, known as partitioning, is a factor of your genetics, age, hormonal profile, metabolism, body composition, diet, recovery, training experience, and training activity. Young, lean, untrained males, with 10 hours of sleep a night, high testosterone levels, and good genetics for muscle building, can have really incredible nutrient partitioning and on a proper training program, they could would add significant lean mass pretty quickly, often times with minimal fat gain, at least at first. As muscle building slows down, extra calories are more likely to be stored as fat. A 45 year old male with multi-year training experience would more than likely see a calorie surplus accumulate as a less than favorable ratio between body fat and lean mass. Moreover, I have seen a lot of individual variability between members of the same demographic, so this one is hard to nail down. The true answer is, "it depends" on a lot of different factors.

Is it better to lift a higher weight to a point of muscle exhaustion or more reps at a lower weight?

This depends on your goals and training program. If you like to train a muscle group or movement more frequently, say, 3 days per week, training to muscular exhaustion would probably be counterproductive, especially as you start handling heavier weights. If you train less frequently, taking reps closer to exhaustion could allow you to work at a higher perceived intensity while taking advantage of the added recovery time between the next session working the same movement or muscle group. As far as using heavier weight vs. lighter weights, keep in mind you can grow from either, albeit through different mechanisms, so your decision would be based on other adaptations, specific to the rep range. Heavier weights are more conducive to strength gain and lighter weights are more conducive to muscular endurance/repeated efforts.

Does drinking a beer or two a few hours after an intense resistance workout reduce the hypertrophic effect of the workout?

To my knowledge, research has yet to look at how low to moderate amounts of alcohol affect protein synthesis post workout. So when these questions come up, I often consider a hypothetical. For example, if you had two twins, both on the same program, diet and rest, one sometimes consumes a beer or two post workout and the other doesn't, who has more muscle in 5 years? To be honest, I wouldn't really expect to see a difference. I can tell you this though, my experience as a coach has shown me that HEAVY drinking is a surefire way to slow gains, mostly because it reliably reduces the intensity of the following workouts. I have not seen the same trend among casual drinkers so I think this is fine.

Why is it that increased muscle mass burns more calories?

Muscle is metabolically active tissue, meaning it uses energy. Growing muscle is also an energy consuming process.

What is the role of protein for exercise?

The primary role of protein in exercise is for the repair and growth of muscular tissue. In most cases, protein (or its building blocks known as amino acids) won't be used as a primary fuel source in resistance training. However, protein will stimulate protein synthesis (muscle building), allowing your body to adapt to the stress you just exposed yourself to, and over time, this results in a larger muscle.

What is a carbohydrate-loading diet?

Carbohydrate loading is a dietary strategy of consuming a high amount of carbohydrates the day or so before prolonged physical activity. Excess carbs will be stored in the muscle tissue as glycogen (fuel for muscle), and this increased fuel storage can be accessed during times of intense and prolonged physical exertion, like distance running. Carb loading is less useful for strength and muscle building purposes because most natural lifters wouldn't be training with an amount of volume that would deplete normal glycogen stores.

What is an anabolic state and why is it important? How does someone create an anabolic state in their body?

For the purposes of building muscle, an anabolic state refers to the state in which your body is "building". Many things trigger this, most important being proper resistance training, rest, and nutrition. Provided you do these things, your body will be in an anabolic state, where it is growing new muscular tissue. However, within 48 hours post workout, this anabolic window will close, the protein synthesis will stop, and muscular tissue will not grow without another bout of resistance training, rest, and nutrition. Over time, the growth from these anabolic phases accumulates and results in a net increase in muscle size.

Contact Info:

Kyle Boggeman

kboggeman@gmail.com

www.sdsctraining.com

9 TAYLOR CARPENTER PERSONAL TRAINING LLC

Charlotte, NC

"Answers Provided by Taylor Carpenter"

Taylor Carpenter Personal Training is a 1 on 1 private personal training studio in Charlotte NC. The only local facility that provides exclusive 1 on 1 training: no groups, no boot camps, no other trainers. Clients benefit from having access to 100% of the training studio during their session. Nutritional guidance is an included service often utilizing MyFitnessPal to learn and track dietary info.

How can someone do resistance training if they don't own weights or belong to a gym?

Everything is technically a resistance exercise, just as everything is technically a cardiorespiratory exercise. If you're 200lbs and you're taking a walk, then you're moving 200lbs...With no weights and no gym access, your primary option will be to do bodyweight movements: squats, lunges, pushups, inverted rows, pull-ups, planks, etc. If you do not have access to a trainer, then there a hundreds of apps and websites to provide workouts and instruction with a quick "Bodyweight Exercise Routine" Google search.

At some point, everyone will need to start amping up the resistance a little bit to avoid a plateau and continue progressing. If you can't afford personal training or higher end gym memberships, then Planet Fitness is $9.99/month, which most people should probably be able to afford. For the average normal gym go-er, they should have everything you need. I often recommend PF to my personal training clients to get extra work.

If someone wants to implement bodyweight exercises into their training program, what's an effective bodyweight workout?

If money is not an issue, you could probably pick up a Jungle Gym XT suspension trainer off of Amazon.com for about $60-$70 and it's durable enough where it should literally last you a lifetime. This is a fun way to implement bodyweight movements into a routine while easily being able progress/regress difficulty based on your angles. I utilize this with all clients: young/old/, overweight/underweight, experienced/inexperienced, etc... If the suspension trainer is not an option, then you would still be looking at plank variations, squats, pushups, inverted rows, supermans, and to increase difficulty, holding isometrics may be your best bet.

Is it true that muscle will turn into fat if someone stops working out?

No. Muscle and fat are two different types of body mass. However, the muscle someone will build from working out will most likely atrophy when they no longer work out regularly leading towards a higher body fat percentage.

Is it safe to work out first thing in the morning on an empty stomach?

Sure, it's safe, but I would not say it's the most efficient way to go about doing things. Whenever you work out, you need to be properly fueled and an empty stomach is not the adequate fuel. Even with the best intentions, a person on an empty stomach will not get as much out of their efforts as someone who is fueled with a healthy plate of carbs pre/intra workout to provide them with some energy. Weight loss and weight gain is a result of calories in vs. calories out. Working out on an empty stomach simply makes life more difficult and workouts less productive.

What is a medical release and when is it necessary?

I have all clients sign a waiver form/amendment clause as all the gyms probably do. It's an understanding that you're participating in a physical activity and the trainer/gym needs to be made aware of any pre-existing injuries or conditions that exist that may deem certain types of exercises harmful. All participants should be thorough and honest when discussing their medical history. Medical releases from doctors should provide the client and trainer with specific guidelines to follow when exercise is allowed coming off a surgery or any negative medical condition that could be made worse with certain types of exercise, such as heart conditions, pregnancy, asthma, etc... I have an additional prenatal exercise release as the different stages of pregnancy provide different limitations to exercise.

How should the diet of someone who's looking to build muscle differ from the diet of someone who's looking to lose weight?

Simple, a calorie surplus is ideal for putting on body mass. A calorie deficit is ideal for losing body mass. With proper macronutrient rationing and progressive heavy loaded resistance exercise, muscle is built.

When it comes to building muscle mass, there seems to be a lot of conflicting information out there. How can people know what advice is good and what is not?

Honestly, the only way to really KNOW would be to cite unbiased scientific journals/studies. Alternatively, you may find sources you trust that have already done the research for you. The average non-fitness professional that's just going to Google a question can't really KNOW for sure the information they're receiving is correct unless they do some research themselves. As with other industries, I usually start with a Google search and seek companies/people with a lot of reviews online. That is probably the best place to start for most people.

Is it true that genetics or body physiology make it impossible for some people to build muscle?

I wouldn't say that's a 100% false. I'm sure there are plenty of medical conditions that make hypertrophy next to impossible. I would say building muscle should be a realistic accomplishment for the vast majority of generally healthy individuals though.

How can people prevent joint injuries or sore joints when lifting weights?

In order: Proper nutrition, adequate sleep, significant warm-up, and excellent form. When you really push yourself with some heavy weights, you'll probably deal with some sore joints and some minor injuries here and there over the years, but if those four things up top are addressed, people really shouldn't deal with too many injuries.

What are the exercises available to build the muscles in the upper body without lifting weights?

Pushups and pull-ups, plus any and all of their variations are going to be the most effective and the foundation of any bodyweight routine.

How to build the lower body without weights?

Squat and lunge variations, to get more glute and hamstring work, single leg hip thrusts are fairly effective. Running and jumping are also lower body resistance moves, but I truly believe that nothing really beats weight training. You can find some dirt cheap dumbbells on Craigslist or, like I said before, the $9 Planet Fitness memberships can probably give you everything you need.

What are some questions people should ask a personal trainer before hiring them?

People should do their research online; seek out reviews from other clients. I would ask about credentials, added nutrition services/advice, pricing, scheduling, policies, etc. Results are mediocre with no nutritional adjustments. I would also ask about the facility you would be getting trained in and how long the trainer has been working in this location. The personal training industry has a very high turnover rate so I would look for some experience and longevity.

Contact Info:
Taylor Carpenter
http://www.taylorcarpenter-pt.com
http://www.facebook.com/charlottetrainer
taylorcarpenter@gmail.com

10 AUM TRAINING CENTER LLC

Boston, MA

"Answers Provided by Chris Carreiro"

Aum Training Center is Boston's only functional medical doctor and personal trainer "w"holistic team. We specialize in helping people radically transform their bodies by offering world-class personal training and advanced metabolic testing. The unique resources we offer uncover all the underlying things holding people back from feeling and looking their best. Through hormone, nutrient, and food allergy testing, along with a comprehensive movement screen and state of the art body composition analysis (BIA), we're able to build a personalized plan for each person based upon their unique biochemistry to optimize their results!

What are the exercises available to build the back muscles?

A well-designed back workout trains all the major muscles of the back (the four muscles that make up the bulk of the back are the Trapezius, Rhomboids, Latissimus Dorsi, Erector spinae). Like with most muscle groups, there are a lot of back exercises to choose from, but only a handful are necessary to build a strong, powerful looking back.

The deadlift is the foundation of any solid weight-training program. At our facility, we usually have our members use the hex bar or trap bar for deadlifting because it doesn't require as much hip and ankle mobility as the standard deadlift. It also places less shearing force on the spine. The hex bar deadlift allows you to lift more weight than the conventional deadlift, which makes it a very effective exercise for packing muscle onto your frame.

The barbell, T-bar row, and seated row are staples in a well-designed back training program because they work everything, from the erector spinae all the way to the trapezius.

The wide-grip pull-up is one of the best exercises you can do to build the middle of your back and your latissimus dorsi.

What are the factors that affect the duration of building the body muscles?

There are multiple factors that affect the amount of time it takes to build muscle.

Progressive Overload

An individual's training experience is a big factor in how long it takes to build muscle. A beginner who is completely new to weight training will see results faster (the initial changes are neurological adaptations) than a seasoned veteran who has been lifting weights for years. The reason is this: a beginner doesn't need to train to momentary failure to create enough stimulus for muscle growth. An experienced lifter, on the other hand, needs to manipulate several variables (see below) in order to overload the muscle to increase the level of tension imposed in order to elicit increases in size. This is known as the overload principle. The main takeaway: changes in your body and muscle size occur through providing progressive overload by manipulating training variables, such as repetition range, number of sets, tempo, length of rest periods, frequency of training, and specific exercise selection. These parameters all influence the length of time and the type of results an individual will achieve in building muscle.

With all this said, one of the main factors that influences all other loading parameters is the number of repetitions. If you're seeking to increase muscle size, researchers have found that you should primarily focus on choosing a weight you can lift (with proper form) between 6 and 12 repetitions. I use the word primarily because, as someone becomes a more advanced lifter, he or she may need to perform sets of fewer repetitions (3-5) in order to overload the muscles enough to create change. This is known as the overload principle: your muscles will only get bigger and stronger if they are forced to adapt to progressive overload.

Nutrition

Nutrition plays a key role in optimizing your body's ability to build muscle. Every individual is different and therefore has different nutritional needs. With that said, a sound principle to follow is building your meals around lean proteins, quality fats, and complex carbohydrates which provide the building blocks your body needs to increase muscle size.

Recovery

Recovery is as important as anything else; you need to give your body the time and resources to actually build new muscle. This means getting at least 7-8 hours of sleep.

What type of cardio should someone do that won't hinder building muscle?

To burn fat without losing muscle, you'd be hard-pressed to do something more effective than sprinting. Sprinters have some of the most muscular physiques you'll find. A study conducted by Phil Campbell and his colleagues showed that 8 sprint intervals with a rest between each sprint increased human growth hormone levels by an average of 771%! After 8 weeks, the average body fat lost was 31%.

Ultimately, the number of sets, reps, intervals, etc are based upon your fitness level. Because sprinting can be very taxing on your nervous system, I recommend sprinting once every 7 days to allow for full recovery.

What are the major steps to building your body muscles?

One of the keys is to focus on compound, multi-joint movement, lifting weights in the 80% to 85% of 1RM. Progressively overloading your body by manipulating training variables, such as repetition range, number of sets, tempo, length of rest periods, frequency of training and specific exercise selection is an art-form and is key for long-term gains in muscle size and strength.

Are food supplements necessary to building muscle?

I'm a believer in eating a whole-food, nutrient-dense food plan first and foremost. I don't think it is imperative to consume supplements to build muscle. However, there are well-researched supplements, such as creatine and glutamine that undoubtedly help accelerate progress.

How much rest should a person take between sets and what is its importance?

The rest interval is very important because it: regulates the partial or nearly complete restoration of the energy substrates needed for maximal performance; allows for the clearance of metabolic waste; allows the central nervous system to recover; slows down the elevated metabolic and heart rates; impacts which hormones are secreted in response to the training. The amount of rest taken between sets is determined by the individual's goal. Sport scientists recommend rest intervals of 3-4 minutes (and even up to 5 minutes) when training with maximal loads: 1-5-rep maximum at 85-100 percent of max. A bodybuilder may choose to go with an incomplete recovery in order to increase the levels of the growth hormone and lactic acid (to enhance hypertrophy). Tolerance to shorter rest intervals happens after years of training. The most important principle to consider about rest intervals and how they impact bodybuilding is that there is an inverse relationship between reps and sets: the more reps you perform, the lighter weights you use and the less rest you need.

How fast or slow should someone perform the reps?

First and foremost, the answer to this question goes back to the individual's goal. A couple of studies from 1989 showed great value in varying the speed of contraction through a training program. With that said, to develop maximal strength, slow-speed training with heavy weights has been shown to have an advantage over high-speed lifting. In order to develop maximum muscle mass, the optimal time that a muscle should contract during a set should be between 20-70 seconds.

How do you train with high volume and medium intensity?

You must optimize recovery through 7-8 hours of sleep each night in addition to consuming a nutrient dense eating plan and consistent soft tissue work (self-myofascial release, foam rolling). Ultimately, you must listen to your body to determine the frequency it can handle in regards to training. If you're constantly getting sick or you're extremely fatigued on a regular basis, perhaps you're exceeding your means. On the other hand, if you're sleeping and eating well and making consistent gains, perhaps you've found just the right dosage of training to reach your goals.

What workouts can be done to build a thicker, wider back?

Focus on progressing the specific exercises I referenced earlier for building a thick, wide back (deadlifts, wide-grip pull-ups).

How does a fitness trainer decide what program is right for their client?

We initially conduct a thorough assessment with every new member, which includes a movement screen, postural assessment, fitness test, review of medical and injury history in addition to thoroughly listening to each person's goals in order to design the best program for him or her.

Contact Info:

Chris Carreiro

Email: coachcarreiro@gmail.com

Call: 774-222-2318

Visit aumtrainingcenter.com

CONCLUSION

Congratulations on making it to the end of this book! We hope that you realize and appreciate the immense level of real world knowledge that you've just acquired. The one thing you may be feeling, at this point, is a bit of "information overload", due to the many tips, pieces of advice, and strategies that are jammed into this book. If you are feeling a bit overwhelmed from everything you've just learned, allow us to offer you one final piece of advice: Take a day to let your brain absorb all of the information you just learned. As they say: "Sleep on it". If you attempt to try and remember and implement everything you just learned, your efforts may tend to be scattered and a bit unorganized. Instead, take a day off from the information. If you do this, you're likely to find that you develop a sense of clarity and a better perspective on the information.

Once you've taken a day to allow yourself to re-focus in this way, we encourage you to slowly go back through the book, writing down the actionable information that you intend to implement. Simply reading and understanding the information is not enough. By writing down the information that you plan on implementing, it will allow you to put a clear plan of action into place for yourself.

As you go through the information, don't worry about the order in which you write things down. The first thing to do is to just get the information down on paper. There are many great strategies and tips within this book, but the goal here is for you to extract the exact advice that you will be taking action on. Don't worry if you are unsure about whether or not you will be taking immediate action on certain advice. Just write down everything that you may possibly take action on.

Once you've compiled this list of action steps and "maybe action steps", begin to prioritize this list. In other words, re-write the list with the actions that you know you're going to take at the top of the list and the action items that you may not take action on towards the bottom of the list. By organizing your list in this way, you will be able to build a practical, useable to-do list, from the information you learned in this book. Once you've done this, you will be in an excellent position to start taking focused steps, with clarity and purpose.

We encourage you to start implementing what you just learned in this book! Just as we have shared interviews with real world experts who actually do what they talk about in this book, it is our hope that you, as the reader, will take real world action on the information you've learned here.

Wishing you all the best in your action-taking, fitness and nutrition endeavors!

www.ingramcontent.com/pod-product-compliance
Lightning Source LLC
Chambersburg PA
CBHW060633290526
45793CB00001B/235